MW00469904

International College of Integrative Manual Therapy™ Wellness Series

Dialogues in Contemporary Rehabilitation for Prevention and Care

Ex2

Functional Exercise Program
for Head and Neck Problems

Developed by

Dr. Sharon (Weiselfish) Giammatteo
Dr. Thomas Giammatteo

ANA Publishing
Bloomfield, CT

North Atlantic Books
Berkeley, CA

Ex 2: Functional Exercise Program for Head and Neck Problems

Published by
ANA Publishing
800 Cottage Grove Road, Ste. 211
Bloomfield, Connecticut 06002

North Atlantic Books
P.O Box 12327
Berkeley, California 94712

This book is solely educational and informational in nature. The reader of this book agrees that the reader, author, and publisher have not formed a professional, or any other, relationship. The reader assumes full responsibility for any changes or lack of changes experienced due to the reading of this book. The reader also assumes full responsibility for choosing to do any of the activities mentioned in this book. The author and the publisher are not liable for any use or misuse of the information contained herein.

The educational information in this book is not intended for diagnosis, prescription, determination of function, or treatment of any conditions or diseases or any health disorder whatsoever. Readers and students of this method are advised to have a healthcare professional monitor their health. The information in this book should not be used as a replacement for proper medical care.

Any person with disease, pathologies, or accidents should be under the care of a healthcare professional, and consult with them before doing any activity in this book.

Ex 2: Functional Exercise Program for Head and Neck Problems is sponsored by the Society for the Study of Native Arts and Sciences, a nonprofit educational corporation whose goals are to develop an educational and crosscultural perspective linking various scientific, social, and artistic fields; to nurture a holistic view of arts, sciences, humanities, and healing; and to publish and distribute literature on the relationship of mind, body, and nature.

North Atlantic Books' publications are available through most bookstores. For further information, call 800-337-2665 or visit our website at www.northatlanticbooks.com.

Substantial discounts on bulk quantities are available to corporations, professional associations, and other organizations. For details and discount information, contact our special sales department.

Cover and book design by Ayelet Maida, A/M Studios
Photographs by Thomas Giammatteo
Printed in the United States of America

LIBRARY OF CONGRESS CATALOGING-IN-PUBLICATION DATA

(Weiselfish) Giammatteo, Sharon.
   Functional exercise program for head and neck problems / developed by Sharon (Weiselfish) Giammatteo; edited by Thomas Giammatteo.
      p. cm. (International College of Integrative Manual Therapy wellness series; 2)
   ISBN 1-55643-365-4 (alk. paper)
   1. Head—Diseases—Exercise therapy. 2. Neck—Diseases—Exercise therapy.
   I. Giammatteo, Thomas. II. Series.

RC936 W454 2000
617.5'1062—dc21   00-058236

1 2 3 4 5 6 7 8 9 / 05 04 03 02 01

Contents

Part **1** Exteroception of Tongue and Intra-Oral Cavity **1**

Part **2** Proprioception of Tongue and Intra-Oral Cavity **8**

Part **3** Strengthening of the Tongue Muscles **20**

Part **4** Strengthening of the Lips and Mouth **24**

Part **5** Strengthening of the Nose Muscles **27**

Part **6** Re-education of Smell **34**

Part **7** Re-education of Taste **39**

Part **8** Re-education of Hearing **44**

Part **9** Re-education of Vision **49**

Part **10** Exteroception of Head and Face **59**

Dialogues in Contemporary Rehabilitation **73**

Exercise **1**: damp washcloth
Exercise **2**: damp washcloth
Exercise **7**: hand mirror
Exercise **18**: spoon
Exercise **19**: spoon
Exercise **20**: spoon
Exercise **29**: hand mirror
Exercise **30**: hand mirror
Exercise **31**: hand mirror
Exercise **32**: onion
Exercise **34**: banana
Exercise **35**: garlic
Exercise **36**: orange
Exercise **37**: reading material
Exercise **39**: audio device
Exercise **40**: ear phones, audio device
Exercise **41**: damp washcloth
Exercise **44**: hand mirror
Exercise **45**: damp washcloth
Exercise **52**: tooth brush
Exercise **53**: damp washcloth
Exercise **54**: damp washcloth
Exercise **55**: tennis ball
Exercise **56**: refrigerator

Introduction

This exercise book is meant for all persons, all ages, all problems which are related to the head, neck, and face. The exercises were compiled by Sharon (Weiselfish) Giammatteo, Ph.D., P.T., IMT,C.

During thirty years of clinical research with clients who have face pain, headaches, and neck problems—the results have been good. Face and jaw pain and weakness; swallowing difficulty; neck motion restrictions; ringing in the ear; blurred vision; snoring; drooling; and so many other problems have been affected in a positive manner with these exercises.

Often, people think they are helpless, yet there are options. Often, people do not know of these options and they become hopeless. These exercises are meant to change life styles. These exercises are meant to decrease discomfort, increase strength and endurance, improve movement and help daily living.

Part **1**

Functional Exercise Program
for Exteroception
of Tongue and Intra-Oral Cavity

Exercise **1**

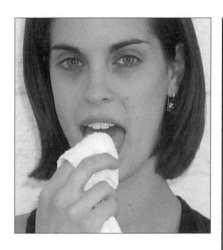

1. Place a damp wash cloth on the tongue.
2. Rub the cloth **gently** on the tongue.
3. Cover the total area of the tongue:
   - Front
   - Back
   - Right side
   - Left side
4. Perform this exercise for 30 seconds.

REPETITIONS: 2

SCHEDULE: 3 times a week for 6 months

BENEFIT: This exercise will improve articulation, speech, swallowing, facial pain. Taste may improve.

Exercise **2**

1. Place a damp wash cloth on the inside of the mouth.
2. Rub the cloth **gently** on the inside of the mouth.
3. Cover the total area of the inside of the mouth:
   - Inside the top lip
   - Inside the bottom lip
   - Right inner cheek
   - Left inner cheek
4. Perform this exercise for 30 seconds.

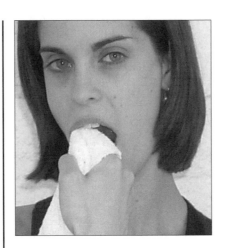

REPETITIONS: 2

SCHEDULE: 3 times a week for 6 months

BENEFIT: This exercise will improve articulation, speech, swallowing, facial pain. Taste may improve.

Exercise **3**

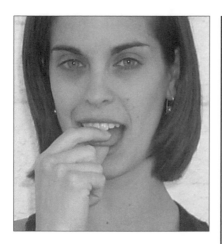

1. Pinch the tongue between the index finger and thumb. **Pinch gently.**
2. Pinch different areas of the tongue:
   - Front
   - Back
   - Right side
   - Left side
3. Perform this exercise for 30 seconds.

REPETITIONS: 1

SCHEDULE: 3 times a week for 6 months

BENEFIT: This exercise will improve articulation, speech, swallowing, facial pain and discomfort of the neck and throat. Taste may improve.

Exercise **4**

1. Pinch the lips between the index finger and thumb. **Pinch gently.**
2. Pinch different areas of the upper and lower lips.
3. Pinch for 30 seconds.

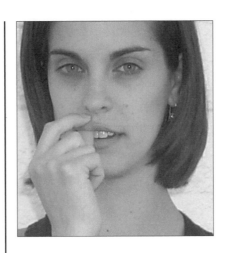

REPETITIONS: 1

SCHEDULE: 3 times a week for 6 months

BENEFIT: This exercise will improve articulation, speech, swallowing, facial pain.

Exercise **5**

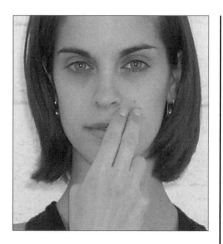

1. Tap the upper and lower lips and the surrounding area (between the nose and the chin, between both cheeks). **Tap gently.**

2. Tap for 30 seconds.

REPETITIONS: 1

SCHEDULE: 3 times a week for 6 months

BENEFIT: This exercise will improve articulation, speech, swallowing, facial pain.

Exercise **6**

1. Scratch the lips and the surrounding area (between the nose and the chin, between both cheeks). **Scratch gently.**
2. Scratch for 30 seconds.

REPETITIONS: 1

SCHEDULE: 3 times a week for 6 months

BENEFIT: This exercise will improve articulation, speech, swallowing, facial pain.

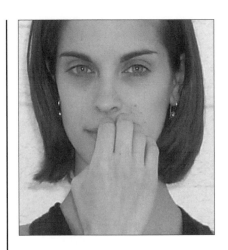

Part **2**

Functional Exercise Program
To Improve Proprioception
of Tongue and Intra-Oral Cavity

Exercise **7**

Stand in front of a mirror.

1. Open your mouth.
2. Stick your tongue out of your mouth:

   - Lift the tip of the tongue up towards your nose. **(A)**

   - Lower the tip of the tongue towards your chin. **(B)**

   - Move the tip of the tongue towards the right cheek. **(C)**

   - Move the tip of the tongue towards the left cheek. **(D)**

3. Bring the tongue back into your mouth.
4. Close your lips firmly.

REPETITIONS: 4

SCHEDULE: 3 times a week for 6 months

BENEFIT: This exercise will improve articulation, speech, swallowing, facial pain and discomfort of the neck and throat.

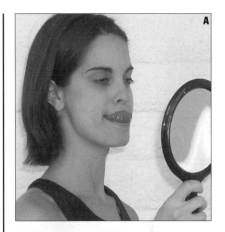

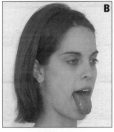

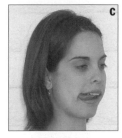

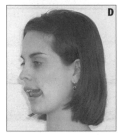

Exercise **8**

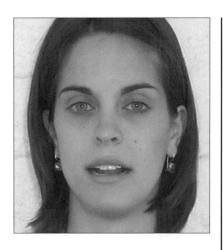

1. Place the tip of the tongue onto the roof of the mouth.
2. Touch the palate just behind the upper teeth.
3. Move the tip of the tongue along the length of the upper teeth.
4. Perform this exercise for 30 seconds.

REPETITIONS: 1

SCHEDULE: 3 times a week for 6 months

BENEFIT: This exercise will improve articulation, speech, swallowing, facial pain and discomfort of the neck and throat and gums.

Exercise **9**

1. Place the tip of the tongue up against the inner top lip.
2. Move the tip of the tongue along the length of the inner top lip.
3. Perform this exercise for 30 seconds.

REPETITIONS: 1

SCHEDULE: 3 times a week for 6 months

BENEFIT: This exercise will improve articulation, speech, swallowing, facial pain and discomfort of the neck and throat and gums.

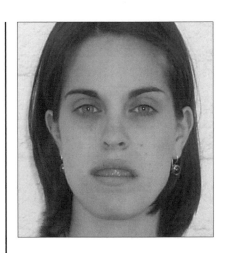

Exercise **10**

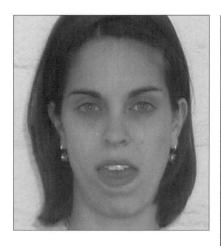

1. Place the tip of the tongue up against the inner lower lip.
2. Move the tip of the tongue along the length of the inner lower lip.
3. Perform this exercise for 30 seconds.

REPETITIONS: 1

SCHEDULE: 3 times a week for 6 months

BENEFIT: This exercise will improve articulation, speech, swallowing, facial pain and discomfort of the neck and throat and gums.

Exercise **11**

1. Place the tip of the tongue on the inner right cheek. **(A)**
2. Move the tip of the tongue around the inner right cheek for 10 seconds.
3. Then place the tip of the tongue on the inner left cheek. **(B)**
4. Move the tip of the tongue around the inner left cheek for 10 seconds.

REPETITIONS: 2

SCHEDULE: 3 times a week for 6 months

BENEFIT: This exercise will improve articulation, speech, swallowing, facial pain and discomfort of the neck and throat and gums.

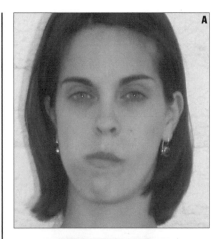

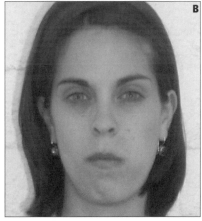

Exercise **12**

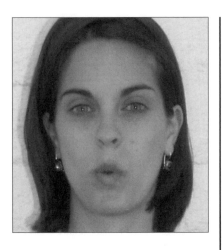

1. Press your upper and lower lips together gently.
2. Then purse your lips. Say out loud: 'O'.
3. Relax.

REPETITIONS: 5

SCHEDULE: 3 times a week for 6 months

BENEFIT: This exercise will improve articulation, speech, swallowing, facial pain and discomfort of the neck and throat.

Exercise **13**

1. Press your upper and lower lips together gently.
2. Keep the lips pressed **gently** together.
3. Attempt to say 'E'.
4. Relax.

REPETITIONS: 5

SCHEDULE: 3 times a week for 6 months

BENEFIT: This exercise will improve articulation, speech, swallowing, facial pain and discomfort of the neck and throat.

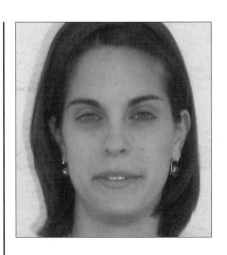

Exercise **14**

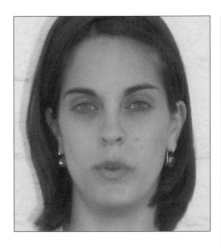

1. Press your upper and lower lips together **gently.**
2. Keep the lips pressed gently together.
3. Attempt to say 'U'.
4. Relax.

REPETITIONS: 5

SCHEDULE: 3 times a week for 6 months

BENEFIT: This exercise will improve articulation, speech, swallowing, facial pain and discomfort of the neck and throat.

Exercise **15**

1. Press your upper and lower lips together **gently.**
2. Keep the lips pressed gently together.
3. Attempt to say 'A'.
4. Relax.

REPETITIONS: 5

SCHEDULE: 3 times a week for 6 months

BENEFIT: This exercise will improve articulation, speech, swallowing, facial pain and discomfort of the neck and throat.

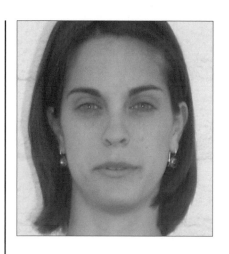

Exercise **16**

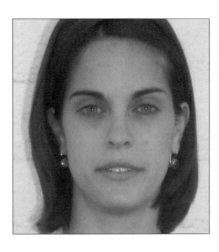

1. Press your upper and lower lips together **gently.**
2. Keep the lips pressed gently together.
3. Attempt to say 'I'.
4. Relax.

REPETITIONS: 5

SCHEDULE: 3 times a week for 6 months

BENEFIT: This exercise will improve articulation, speech, swallowing, facial pain and discomfort of the neck and throat.

Exercise **17**

1. Press your upper and lower lips together **gently.**
2. Keep the lips pressed gently together.
3. Attempt to say 'Y'.
4. Relax.

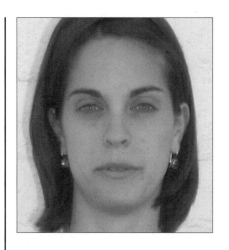

REPETITIONS: 5

SCHEDULE: 3 times a week for 6 months

BENEFIT: This exercise will improve articulation, speech, swallowing, facial pain and discomfort of the neck and throat.

Part **3**

Functional Exercise Program to Improve Strength of the Tongue Muscles

Exercise **18**

1. Place a spoon inside your mouth, on your tongue. (The concave side of the spoon is facing down.)
2. Keep the lips lightly pressed together.
3. Push the convex part of the spoon up towards the palate, with your tongue.
4. Maintain the upwards pressure of the tongue for 30 seconds.

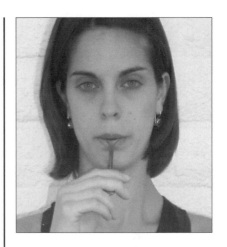

REPETITIONS: 1

SCHEDULE: 3 times a week for 6 months

BENEFIT: This exercise will improve articulation, speech, swallowing, facial pain and discomfort of the neck and throat.

Exercise **19**

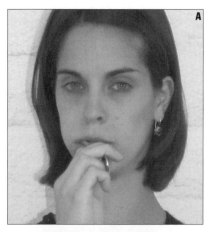

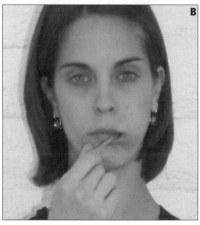

1. Place a spoon inside your mouth, at the right side of your tongue. (The concave side of the spoon is facing towards the tongue.) **(A)**
2. Keep the lips lightly pressed together.
3. Push the spoon against the inner right cheek.
4. Maintain the pressure of the tongue for 30 seconds.
5. Repeat Steps 1–4 for the left cheek. **(B)**

REPETITIONS: 1

SCHEDULE: 3 times a week for 6 months

BENEFIT: This exercise will improve articulation, speech, swallowing, facial pain and discomfort of the neck and throat.

Exercise **20**

1. Place a spoon inside your mouth, on your tongue. (The concave side of the spoon is facing down.)
2. Keep the lips pressed together lightly.
3. Attempt to pull the spoon out of your mouth. (Do not allow the spoon to be pulled out of your mouth.)
4. Maintain the resistance for 30 seconds.

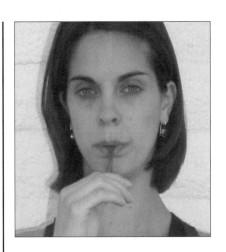

REPETITIONS: 1

SCHEDULE: 3 times a week for 6 months

BENEFIT: This exercise will improve articulation, speech, swallowing, facial pain and discomfort of the neck and throat.

Part **4**

Functional Exercise Program
To Improve Strength
of the Lips and Mouth

Exercise **21**

1. Insert thumb and index finger between your lips.
2. Try to form an 'O' with your lips.
3. Resist the formation of 'O' with thumb and index finger.
4. Maintain the resistance for 30 seconds.

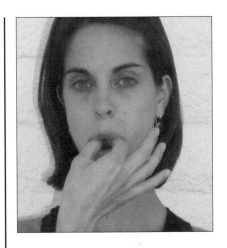

REPETITIONS: 1

SCHEDULE: 3 times a week for 6 months

BENEFIT: This exercise will improve articulation, speech, swallowing, facial pain and discomfort of the neck and throat.

Exercise **22**

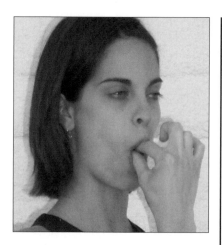

1. Insert thumb and index finger between your lips.
2. Try to press the two lips, upper and lower together.
3. Resist bringing the lips together with your thumb and index finger.
4. Maintain the resistance for 30 seconds.

REPETITIONS: 1

SCHEDULE: 3 times a week for 6 months

BENEFIT: This exercise will improve articulation, speech, swallowing, facial pain and discomfort of the neck and throat.

Part **5**

Functional Exercise Program to Improve Strength of the Nose Muscles

Exercise **23**

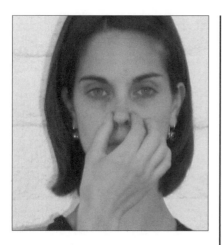

1. Place a thumb and index finger on either side of the nostril.
2. Pinch the nostrils very **gently.**
3. Resist pinching the nostrils, by spreading apart the nostrils apart.
4. Maintain the resistance for 20 seconds.

REPETITIONS: 1

SCHEDULE: 3 times a week for 6 months

BENEFIT: This exercise will improve breathing, and will decrease headaches, facial pain, and neck discomfort. Smell may improve. Allergies and sinus conditions may improve.

Exercise **24**

1. Place a finger tip on the tip of your nose.
2. Without moving your head forward, push the tip of the nose **gently** against your finger tip. (**Do not move your head at all.**)
3. Maintain this isometric resistance for 20 seconds.

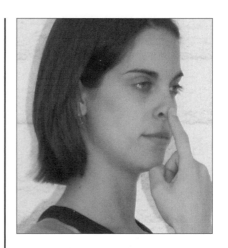

REPETITIONS: 1

SCHEDULE: 3 times a week for 6 months

BENEFIT: This exercise will improve breathing, and will decrease headaches, facial pain, and neck discomfort.

Exercise **25**

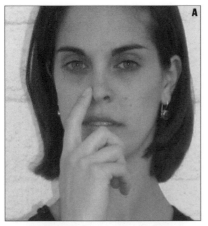

A

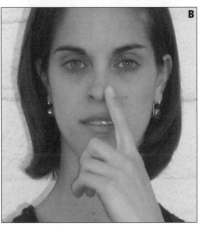

B

1. Place a finger tip on the right side of the tip of your nose. **(A)**
2. Without moving your head, push the tip of your nose against your finger tip. (**Do not move your head at all.**)
3. Maintain this isometric resistance for 20 seconds.
4. Repeat Step 1–3 with the left side of the tip of your nose. **(B)**

REPETITIONS: 1

SCHEDULE: 3 times a week for 6 months

BENEFIT: This exercise will improve breathing, and will decrease headaches, facial pain, and neck discomfort.

Exercise **26**

1. Place a finger tip on the top of the tip of your nose.

2. Without moving your head, attempt to look upwards, pushing your finger tip gently against the top of the tip of your nose. (**Do not move your head at all.**)

3. Maintain this isometric resistance for 20 seconds.

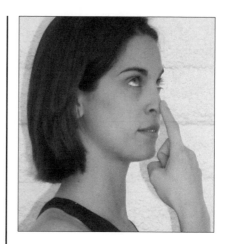

REPETITIONS: 1

SCHEDULE: 3 times a week for 6 months

BENEFIT: This exercise will improve breathing, and will decrease headaches and eye pain, facial pain and neck discomfort.

Exercise **27**

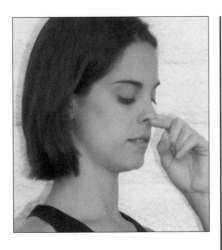

1. Place a finger tip underneath the tip of your nose.

2. Without moving your head, attempt to look down, pushing your finger tip gently against the underside of the tip of your nose. (**Do not move your head at all.**)

3. Maintain this isometric resistance for 20 seconds.

REPETITIONS: 1

SCHEDULE: 3 times a week for 6 months

BENEFIT: This exercise will improve breathing, and will decrease headaches and eye pain, facial pain and neck discomfort.

Exercise **28**

1. Place the index finger on the top of the tip of your nose.

2. Place the thumb under your chin. (**Do not move your face, head or mouth.**)

3. Attempt to open your mouth.

4. Resist mouth opening by gently pressing your thumb against your chin. Keep the index finger on your nose. (**Do not move your head at all.**)

5. Maintain this isometric resistance for 20 seconds

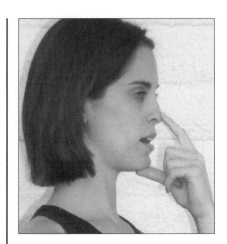

REPETITIONS: 1

SCHEDULE: 3 times a week for 6 months

BENEFIT: This exercise will improve articulation, speech, swallowing, facial pain and discomfort of the neck and throat.

Part **6**

Functional Exercise Program for Re-Education of Smell

Exercise **29**

1. Look at your nostrils in front of a mirror.
2. Insert a finger tip inside your nostril on one side only (insert one millimeter).
3. Breathe in through your nose.
4. Insert a finger tip inside your other nostril (insert one millimeter).
5. Breathe in through your nose.

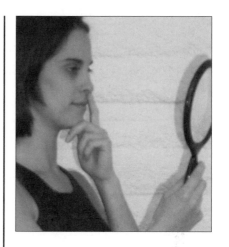

REPETITIONS: 5 per nostril

SCHEDULE: 3 times a week for 6 months

BENEFIT: This exercise will improve breathing and decrease facial pain. Sense of smell may improve.

Exercise **30**

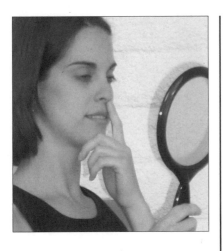

1. Look at your nostrils in front of a mirror.
2. Insert a finger tip inside your nostril on one side only (insert one millimeter).
3. Blow out through your nose.
4. Insert a finger tip inside your other nostril (insert one millimeter).
5. Blow out through your nose.

REPETITIONS: 5 per nostril

SCHEDULE: 3 times a week for 6 months

BENEFIT: This exercise will improve breathing and decrease facial pain. Sense of smell may improve.

Exercise **31**

1. Look at a mirror.
2. Breathe from your nose onto the mirror until you can produce a 'fog' on the mirror.

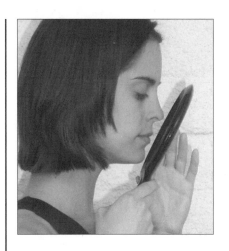

REPETITIONS: 1

SCHEDULE: 3 times a week for 6 months

BENEFIT: This exercise will improve breathing and decrease facial pain. Sense of smell may improve.

Exercise **32**

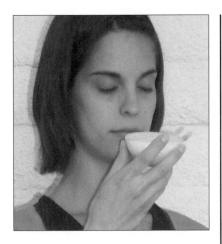

1. Take an onion.
2. Peel the onion.
3. Close your eyes.
4. Hold the onion 2 inches from your nose.
5. Breathe in through your nose.

REPETITIONS: 5

SCHEDULE: 3 times a week for 6 months

BENEFIT: This exercise will improve breathing and decrease facial pain. Sense of smell may improve.

Part **7**

Functional Exercise Program for Re-education of Taste

Exercise **33**

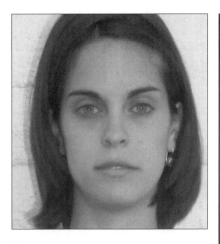

1. Place your complete tongue up against the palate.
2. Relax your jaw.
3. Breathe through your nose.
4. Press the tongue upwards, against the palate.
5. The tongue is barely touching the back of the top teeth.
6. Relax the tongue.

REPETITIONS: 5

SCHEDULE: 3 times a week for 6 months

BENEFIT: This exercise will improve articulation, speech, swallowing, facial pain and discomfort of the neck and throat.

Exercise **34**

1. Place a banana on your tongue. (The whole banana, as far back as it will go without causing you to gag.)
2. Relax your jaw.
3. Breathe through your nose.
4. Press the tongue upwards, against the palate, so that the banana is 'squished'.
5. Keep the upwards pressure on the banana for 30 seconds.
6. Relax.

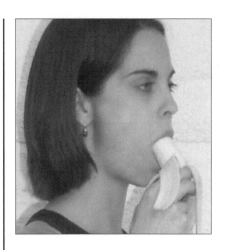

REPETITIONS: 1

SCHEDULE: 3 times a week for 6 months

BENEFIT: This exercise will improve articulation, speech, swallowing, facial pain and discomfort of the neck and throat. Taste may improve.

Exercise 35

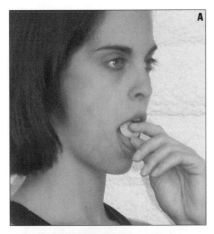

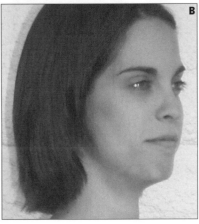

1. Take a clove of garlic.
2. Place the clove of garlic on the front part (not the tip) of your tongue. **(A)**
3. Relax your jaw.
4. Breathe through your nose.
5. Press the tongue upwards, against the palate, so that the garlic is 'squished.' **(B)**
6. Keep the upwards pressure on the garlic for 30 seconds.
7. Relax.

REPETITIONS: 1

SCHEDULE: 3 times a week for 6 months

BENEFIT: This exercise will improve articulation, speech, swallowing, facial pain and discomfort of the neck and throat. Taste may improve.

Exercise **36**

1. Take a piece of orange.
2. Place the piece of orange on the front part (not the tip) of your tongue. **(A)**
3. Relax your jaw.
4. Breathe through your nose.
5. Press the tongue upwards, against the palate, so that the orange is 'squished'.**(B)**
6. Keep the upwards pressure on the orange for 30 seconds.
7. Relax.

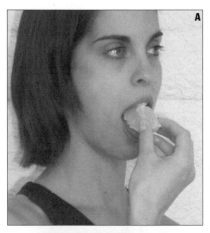

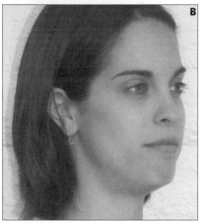

REPETITIONS: 1

SCHEDULE: 3 times a week for 6 months

BENEFIT: This exercise will improve articulation, speech, swallowing, facial pain and discomfort of the neck and throat. Taste may improve.

Part **8**

Functional Exercise Program
for Re-Education
of Hearing

Complimentary Approach

There is a Tomasi process to re-educate higher and lower end frequency hearing.

This process may decrease discomfort from background noises

Exercise **37**

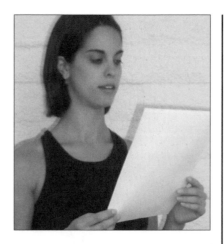

Practice talking out loud.

1. Write down a paragraph of 100 words.
2. Read out loud in a low voice. (**Listen carefully to your own voice.**)
3. Read out loud in a loud voice. (**Listen carefully to your own voice.**)
4. Shout out loud. (**Listen carefully to your own voice.**)

REPETITIONS: 1

SCHEDULE: 3 times a week for 6 months

BENEFIT: This exercise will improve concentration and attention span. Hearing may improve.

Exercise **38**

1. Tap on your ear while you listen to the television, radio, tape recorder, CD, etc.

2. Use three fingers (index, third and fourth fingers) and tap on the outer portion of your ear.

   - Support your arm so that you will not be fatigued.

   - It is important to perform this exercise on both sides (both ears).

   - It is acceptable if someone else taps lightly on your ear.

3. Perform this exercise for at least 5 minutes at a time.

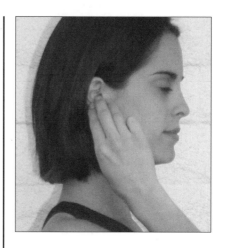

REPETITIONS: 1

SCHEDULE: 3 times a week for 6 months

BENEFIT: This exercise will decrease ear sounds, facial, head and neck discomfort. Hearing may improve.

Exercise **39**

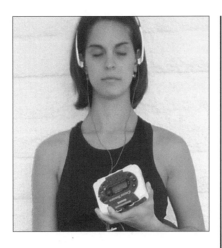

1. Use ear phones. Listen to the radio. (Not to music.)
2. Focus. Concentrate on listening to the words for at least 5 minutes.
3. Play the radio as low as you can hear it, so that it is not any louder than it need be.
4. Close your eyes during this exercise.

REPETITIONS: 1

SCHEDULE: 3 times a week for 6 months

BENEFIT: This exercise will improve concentration and attention span. Hearing may improve.

Part **9**

Functional Exercise Program
for Re-Education
of Vision

Complimentary Approach

An exceptional program for restoration of vision is Meir Schneider's work. Read *Self-Healing, My Life and My Vision,* and *Handbook for Self-Healing* by Meir Schneider.

This process has exceptional results of improved vision for even severe visually impaired persons.

Exercise **40**

1. Take a warm, damp towel. (Be sure that the towel is clean.)
2. Place the towel lightly over your OPENED eyes. Look into the towel for 1 minute.

REPETITIONS: 1

SCHEDULE: 3 times a week for 6 months

BENEFIT: This exercise will decrease eye pain and improve visual clarity. Head, face and neck discomfort will be reduced.

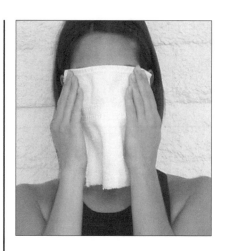

Exercise **41**

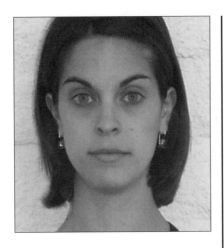

1. Shut off all lights in the room. (The room should be dark.)
2. Open your eyes. Try to force your eyes open (NOT using your hands!).
3. Look into the dark for 1 minute.

REPETITIONS: 1

SCHEDULE: 3 times a week for 6 months

BENEFIT: This exercise will decrease eye pain and improve visual clarity. Head, face and neck discomfort will be reduced.

Exercise **42**

1. Look at yourself in a mirror.
2. Force your eyes open wide. (NOT using your hands!)
3. Look into your own eyes for 1 minute.

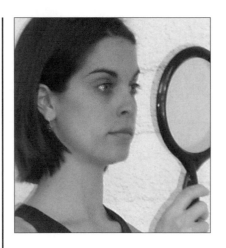

REPETITIONS: 1

SCHEDULE: 3 times a week for 6 months

BENEFIT: This exercise will decrease eye pain and improve visual clarity. Head, face and neck discomfort will be reduced.

Exercise **43**

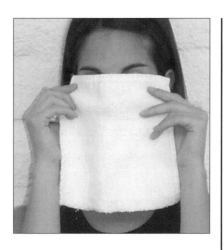

1. Place a towel over your eyes.
2. Do not move your head or neck.
3. Attempt to push away the towel with your eyes. Do not succeed in moving the towel.
4. Perform this exercise for 1 minute.

REPETITIONS: 1

SCHEDULE: 3 times a week for 6 months

BENEFIT: This exercise will decrease eye pain and improve visual clarity. Head, face and neck discomfort will be reduced.

Exercise **44**

1. Place a thumb and index finger of one hand onto your eyes, with the eyelids closed.
2. **VERY GENTLY** keep your eyelids closed, while you attempt to open your eyelids.
3. Do not succeed in opening your eyelids.
4. Perform this exercise for 1 minute.

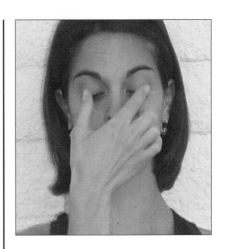

REPETITIONS: 1

SCHEDULE: 3 times a week for 6 months

BENEFIT: This exercise will decrease eye pain and improve visual clarity. Head, face and neck discomfort will be reduced.

Exercise **45**

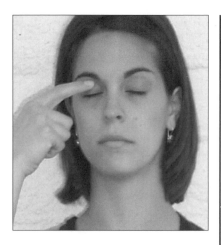

1. With your eyes closed, place a finger tip lightly on the top part of the eyeball.
2. Attempt to look up.
3. Resist the movement of the eyeball with your finger tip. **Resist gently!**
4. Repeat exercise for other eye.

REPETITIONS: 5

SCHEDULE: 3 times a week for 6 months

BENEFIT: This exercise will decrease eye pain and improve visual clarity. Head, face and neck discomfort will be reduced.

Exercise **46**

1. With your eyes closed, place a finger tip lightly on the right side of your right eyeball. **(A)**
2. Attempt to look to the right.
3. Resist the movement of the eyeball with your finger tip. **Resist gently!**
4. Repeat exercise for your left eye, looking left. **(B)**

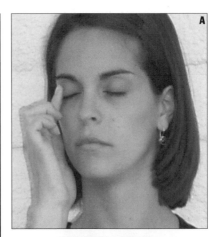

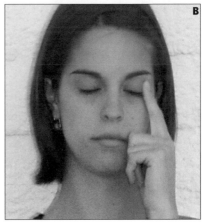

REPETITIONS: 5

SCHEDULE: 3 times a week for 6 months

BENEFIT: This exercise will decrease eye pain and improve visual clarity. Head, face and neck discomfort will be reduced.

Exercise **47**

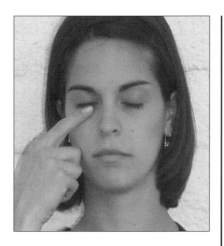

1. With your eyes closed, place a finger tip lightly on the bottom part of the eyeball.
2. Attempt to look down.
3. Resist the movement of the eyeball with your finger tip. **Resist gently!**
4. Repeat exercise for other eye.

REPETITIONS: 5

SCHEDULE: 3 times a week for 6 months

BENEFIT: This exercise will decrease eye pain and improve visual clarity. Head, face and neck discomfort will be reduced.

Part **10**

Functional Exercise Program to Improve Exteroception of Head and Face

Exercise **48**

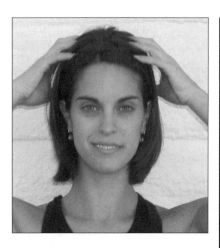

1. Rub your scalp over dry hair.
2. Rub lightly.
3. Rub harder.
4. Rub all areas of the head.
5. Perform exercise for 3 minutes.

REPETITIONS: 1

SCHEDULE: 3 times a week for 6 months

BENEFIT: This exercise will decrease head swelling and discomfort.

Exercise **49**

1. Rub your face.
2. Rub lightly.
3. Rub harder.
4. Rub all areas of the face.
5. Perform exercise for 3 minutes.

REPETITIONS: 1

SCHEDULE: 3 times a week for 6 months

BENEFIT: This exercise will decrease facial pain and discomfort.

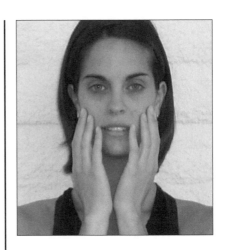

Exercise **50**

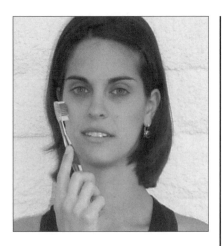

1. Take a 'soft' bristle toothbrush (not medium or hard).
2. Brush the face in 2 directions:
   - up and down
   - right and left
3. Brush the whole face.
4. Perform exercise for 3 minutes.

REPETITIONS: 1

SCHEDULE: 3 times a week for 6 months

BENEFIT: This exercise will decrease facial pain and discomfort. Normal sensory awareness of the face will improve.

Exercise **51**

1. Take a warm, damp cloth. (It should not be cold or hot, or wet.)
2. Place the cloth over the face with your eyes closed.
3. Keep the cloth over your face for 30 seconds.

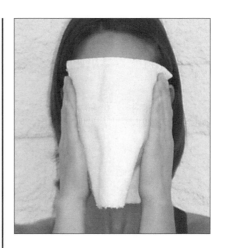

REPETITIONS: 1

SCHEDULE: 3 times a week for 6 months

BENEFIT: This exercise will decrease facial pain and discomfort.

Exercise **52**

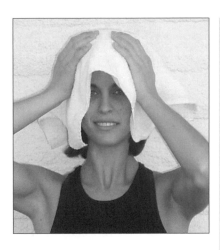

1. Take a warm, damp cloth. (It should not be cold or hot, or wet.)
2. Place the cloth over the head.
3. Keep the cloth over your head for 30 seconds.

REPETITIONS: 1

SCHEDULE: 3 times a week for 6 months

BENEFIT: This exercise will decrease head discomfort.

Exercise **53**

1. Take a tennis ball.
2. Press it against all aspects of your head and face.
3. Press lightly.
4. Perform the exercise for 1 minute.

REPETITIONS: 1

SCHEDULE: 3 times a week for 6 months

BENEFIT: This exercise will decrease facial pain and discomfort. Normal sensory awareness of the face will improve.

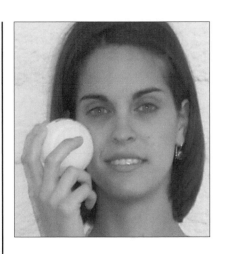

Exercise **54**

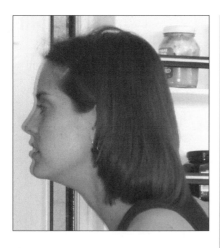

1. Open your refrigerator.
2. Put your face and head inside the refrigerator.
3. Breathe in through your nose.
4. Keep your eyes closed.
5. Keep your face and head in the refrigerator for 30 seconds.

REPETITIONS: 1

SCHEDULE: 3 times a week for 6 months

BENEFIT: This exercise will decrease facial pain and discomfort. Normal sensory awareness of the face will improve. Temperature of the face will improve.

Exercise **55**

1. Sit up with your chin tucked in, your jaw relaxed, breathing through your nose.

2. Place a hand against the right side of your head. (**Do not move your head and neck.**) **(A)**

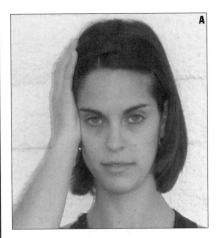

3. Push your hand against the right side of your head; push your head against your hand. **Resist gently!**

4. Maintain the resistance for 20 seconds.

5. Repeat Steps 1–4 with left side. **(B)**

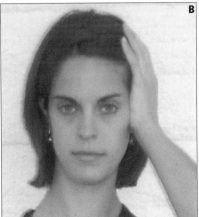

REPETITIONS: 1

SCHEDULE: 3 times a week for 6 months

BENEFIT: This exercise will improve face and head strength. Discomfort of the face, head and neck will decrease.

Exercise **56**

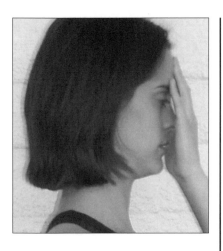

1. Sit up with your chin tucked in, your jaw relaxed, breathing through your nose.
2. Place a hand against your forehead. (**Do not move your head and neck.**)
3. Push your hand against your forehead; push your head against your hand. **Resist gently!**
4. Maintain the resistance for 20 seconds.

REPETITIONS: 1

SCHEDULE: 3 times a week for 6 months

BENEFIT: This exercise will improve face and head strength. Discomfort of the face, head and neck will decrease.

Exercise **57**

1. Sit up with your chin tucked in, your jaw relaxed, breathing through your nose.
2. Place a hand against the back of your head. (**Do not move your head and neck.**)
3. Push your hand against the back of your head; push your head against your hand. **Resist gently!**
4. Maintain the resistance for 20 seconds.

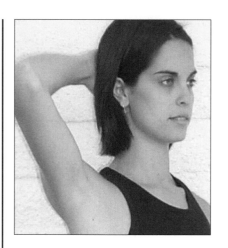

REPETITIONS: 1

SCHEDULE: 3 times a week for 6 months

BENEFIT: This exercise will improve face and head strength. Discomfort of the face, head and neck will decrease.

Exercise **58**

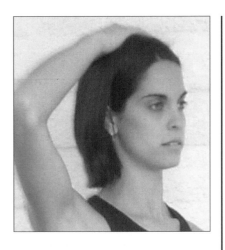

1. Sit up with your chin tucked in, your jaw relaxed, breathing through your nose.
2. Place a hand on the top of your head.
3. Attempt to push upwards, against your hand. Your hand will push lightly onto the top of the head. **Resist gently!**
4. Maintain the resistance for 20 seconds.

REPETITIONS: 1

SCHEDULE: 3 times a week for 6 months

BENEFIT: This exercise will improve face and head strength. Discomfort of the face, head and neck will decrease.

Exercise **59**

1. Sit up with your chin tucked in, your jaw relaxed, breathing through your nose.
2. Place a hand on the right side of your chin. (**Do not move your head, neck or chin.**) **(A)**
3. Push your hand against your chin; push your chin against your hand. **Resist gently!**
4. Maintain the resistance for 20 seconds.
5. Repeat Steps 1–4 with the left side. **(A)**

REPETITIONS: 1

SCHEDULE: 3 times a week for 6 months

BENEFIT: This exercise will improve face, jaw, and head strength. Discomfort of the face, head and neck will decrease.

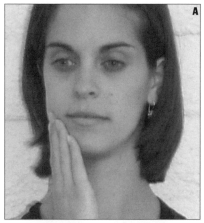

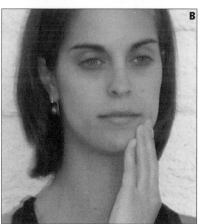

Exercise **60**

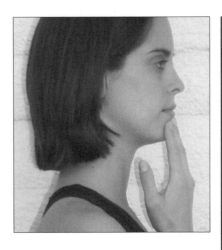

1. Sit up with your chin tucked in, your jaw relaxed, breathing through your nose.
2. Place a hand on the front of your chin. (**Do not move your head, neck or chin.**)
3. Push your hand against your chin; push your chin against your hand. **Resist gently!**
4. Maintain the resistance for 20 seconds.

REPETITIONS: 1

SCHEDULE: 3 times a week for 6 months

BENEFIT: This exercise will improve face, jaw, and head strength. Discomfort of the face, head and neck will decrease.

Dialogues in
Contemporary Rehabilitation

DCR is the company for Integrative Manual Therapy, the Integrated Systems Approach, Integrative Diagnostics, and Functional and Structural Rehabilitation. Founded in the early 1980s by Mary Fiorentino, O.T.,R. Sharon (Weiselfish) Giammatteo initiated a transformation in the educational process incorporated by DCR in 1986, when she received ownership from Mary. Faculty of DCR are trained in all areas of manual therapy; they are experts in the fields of orthopedics and sports medicine, chronic pain, neuro-rehabilitation, pediatrics, geriatrics, women's and men's health issues, cardiopulmonary rehabilitation, and more. Almost 100 percent of the material offered by DCR has been developed, research and present-day results performed, at Regional Physical Therapy in Connecticut.

DCR MISSION STATEMENT

DCR offers hope, practice and purpose. Our goal is recovery; our intention is learning, teaching, and understanding. Our field of accomplishment is extended to client, family, community and world. We accept tomorrow's knowledge as today's quest. We are not hindered by greed, inhibitions, or belief systems. We are multi-denominational, cross-cultural, and non-racial in orientation. We wish to facilitate recovery from dysfunction through growth and development.

Biomechanics with: Muscle Energy and 'Beyond' Technique
MET1: Pelvis, Sacrum and Spine
MET2: Upper and Lower Extremities and Rib Cage
MET3: Advanced Biomechanics: Sacrum and Spine
MET4: Type III Biomechanical Dysfunction: Spine and Extremities
and Bone Bruises

Muscle and Circulation with Strain and Counterstrain Technique
SCS1: Strain and Counterstrain for Orthopedics and Neurologic
Patient
SCS2: Advanced Strain and Counterstrain for Autonomic Nervous
System

**Connective Tissue with Myofascial Release, The 3-Planar Fascial
Fulcrum Technique**
MFR1: Myofascial Release for Orthopedic, Neurologic, Geriatric
Patient
MFR2: Myofascial Mapping for Integrative Diagnostics

Peripheral Nerve Tissue Tension: Hypomobility and Fibrosis
NTT2: Neural Tissue Tension Technique

Cranial and the Craniosacral System with: The Cranial Therapy Series
CTS1: Osseous, Suture, Joint and Membrane
CTS2: Membrane, Fluid, Facial Vault and Cranial Gear-Complex
CTS3: Cranial Diaphragm Compression Syndromes; CSF Fluid:
Production, Distribution and Absorption; Immunology
CTS4: Neuronal Regeneration, Cranial Nerves, and
Neurotransmission
CTSA1: Postural Reflexes
CTSA2: Vasculature in the Brain
CTSA3: The Eye

Organs with Visceral Mobilization
VMET1: Visceral Mobilization with Muscle Energy and 'Beyond'—
Focus GI Tract
VMET2: Women's and Men's Health Issues
VMET3: Respiratory Rehabilitation
VMET4: Cardiac Habilitation
VMET5: The Liver

The Lymphatic System
LYM1: Congestion Therapy
LYM2: Immune Preference

Compression Syndromes
COMP1:Compression Syndromes of the Upper Extremities
COMP2:Compression Syndromes of the Lower Extremities
COMP3:Diaphragm Compression Syndromes

Neuro-Rehabilitation
DMT: Developmental Manual Therapy for the Neurologic Patient

Integrative Diagnostics
IDS: Integrative Diagnostic Series: Myofascial Mapping,
Neurofascial Process, Rx Plans
IDAP: Integrative Diagnostics for Applied Psychosynthesis
IDLB: Integrative Diagnostics for Lower Back

Integrative Seminars
IMTS: Integrative Manual Therapy for Neck, Thoracic Outlet,
Shoulder and Upper Extremity
IMTUE/LESM: Integrative Manual Therapy for Upper and Lower
Extremities in Sports Medicine
IMTCCC: Integrative Manual Therapy for Craniocervical,
Craniofacial, Craniomandibular

Functional Rehabilitation
Therapeutic Horizons: The Brain (BANM); The Heart (BACM);
The Pelvis (BANRA); Advanced Levels 1–3 (BAAL1–3)

NES & DCR Offer Adjunct Educational Material in Integrative Manual Therapy

BOOKS

Manual Therapy for the Pelvis, Sacrum, Cervical, Thoracic and Lumbar Spine, with Muscle Energy Technique—A Contemporary Clinical Analysis of Biomechanics by Sharon Weiselfish, Ph.D., P.T.

Integrative Manual Therapy for the Autonomic Nervous System and Related Disorders by Thomas Giammatteo, D.C. P.T., and Sharon (Weiselfish) Giammatteo, Ph.D., P.T.

Integrative Manual Therapy for the Upper and Lower Extremities, Introducing Synergic Pattern Release with Strain and Counterstrain Technique, and Muscle Energy and 'Beyond' Technique for the Peripheral Joints by Sharon (Weiselfish) Giammatteo, Ph.D., P.T., edited by Thomas Giammatteo, D.C., P.T.

By Sharon (Weiselfish) Giammatteo, Ph.D., P.T.
Produced by Northeast Seminars

Muscle Energy Technique Series
#1 Pelvis
#2 Sacrum
#3 Thoracic and Lumbar Spine
#4 Cervical and Thoracic Spine
#5 Strain and Counterstrain for the Orthopedic and Neurologic Patient
#6 Myofascial Release, the 3-Planar Fascial Fulcrum Approach, for the Orthopedic, Neurologic and Geriatric Patient
#7 Advanced Manual Therapy for the Low Back
#8 Integrative Manual Therapy: A Patient in Process
#9 Manual Therapy for the Low Back: Standards for the Health Care Industry for the 21st Century
#10 Muscle Energy and 'Beyond' Technique for the Upper Extremities
#11 Muscle Energy and 'Beyond' Technique for the Lower Extremities

For further information regarding educational products, please contact Northeast Seminars at:

Northeast Seminars
P.O. Box 522
East Hampstead, NH 03826
Tel: 800-272-2044
Fax: 603-329-7045
E-mail: neseminar@aol.com
Website: www.neseminars.com

For further information regarding DCR products and seminars, please contact DCR at:

DCR
Dialogues in Contemporary Rehabilitation
800 Cottage Grove Road, Suite 211
Bloomfield, CT 06002
Tel: 860-243-5220
Fax: 860-243-5304
E-mail: dcrhealth@aol.com
Website: www.dcrhealth.com

Exercise Program

PATIENT NAME _____ DATE _____

HEALTHCARE PRACTITIONER _____ PHONE _____

6 MONTH SESSION BEGINS _____

SESSION FREQUENCY: ☐ Daily   ☐ 3 times a week

Perform the following exercises for 30 minutes per session.
Follow specific instructions for each exercise.

☐ Exercise **1**	☐ Exercise **21**	☐ Exercise **41**
☐ Exercise **2**	☐ Exercise **22**	☐ Exercise **42**
☐ Exercise **3**	☐ Exercise **23**	☐ Exercise **43**
☐ Exercise **4**	☐ Exercise **24**	☐ Exercise **44**
☐ Exercise **5**	☐ Exercise **25**	☐ Exercise **45**
☐ Exercise **6**	☐ Exercise **26**	☐ Exercise **46**
☐ Exercise **7**	☐ Exercise **27**	☐ Exercise **47**
☐ Exercise **8**	☐ Exercise **28**	☐ Exercise **48**
☐ Exercise **9**	☐ Exercise **29**	☐ Exercise **49**
☐ Exercise **10**	☐ Exercise **30**	☐ Exercise **50**
☐ Exercise **11**	☐ Exercise **31**	☐ Exercise **51**
☐ Exercise **12**	☐ Exercise **32**	☐ Exercise **52**
☐ Exercise **13**	☐ Exercise **33**	☐ Exercise **53**
☐ Exercise **14**	☐ Exercise **34**	☐ Exercise **54**
☐ Exercise **15**	☐ Exercise **35**	☐ Exercise **55**
☐ Exercise **16**	☐ Exercise **36**	☐ Exercise **56**
☐ Exercise **17**	☐ Exercise **37**	☐ Exercise **57**
☐ Exercise **18**	☐ Exercise **38**	☐ Exercise **58**
☐ Exercise **19**	☐ Exercise **39**	☐ Exercise **59**
☐ Exercise **20**	☐ Exercise **40**	☐ Exercise **60**

Notes

Exercise Program

PATIENT NAME _____ DATE _____

HEALTHCARE PRACTITIONER _____ PHONE _____

6 MONTH SESSION BEGINS _____

SESSION FREQUENCY: ☐ Daily ☐ 3 times a week

Perform the following exercises for 30 minutes per session.
Follow specific instructions for each exercise.

☐ Exercise **1**	☐ Exercise **21**	☐ Exercise **41**
☐ Exercise **2**	☐ Exercise **22**	☐ Exercise **42**
☐ Exercise **3**	☐ Exercise **23**	☐ Exercise **43**
☐ Exercise **4**	☐ Exercise **24**	☐ Exercise **44**
☐ Exercise **5**	☐ Exercise **25**	☐ Exercise **45**
☐ Exercise **6**	☐ Exercise **26**	☐ Exercise **46**
☐ Exercise **7**	☐ Exercise **27**	☐ Exercise **47**
☐ Exercise **8**	☐ Exercise **28**	☐ Exercise **48**
☐ Exercise **9**	☐ Exercise **29**	☐ Exercise **49**
☐ Exercise **10**	☐ Exercise **30**	☐ Exercise **50**
☐ Exercise **11**	☐ Exercise **31**	☐ Exercise **51**
☐ Exercise **12**	☐ Exercise **32**	☐ Exercise **52**
☐ Exercise **13**	☐ Exercise **33**	☐ Exercise **53**
☐ Exercise **14**	☐ Exercise **34**	☐ Exercise **54**
☐ Exercise **15**	☐ Exercise **35**	☐ Exercise **55**
☐ Exercise **16**	☐ Exercise **36**	☐ Exercise **56**
☐ Exercise **17**	☐ Exercise **37**	☐ Exercise **57**
☐ Exercise **18**	☐ Exercise **38**	☐ Exercise **58**
☐ Exercise **19**	☐ Exercise **39**	☐ Exercise **59**
☐ Exercise **20**	☐ Exercise **40**	☐ Exercise **60**

Notes